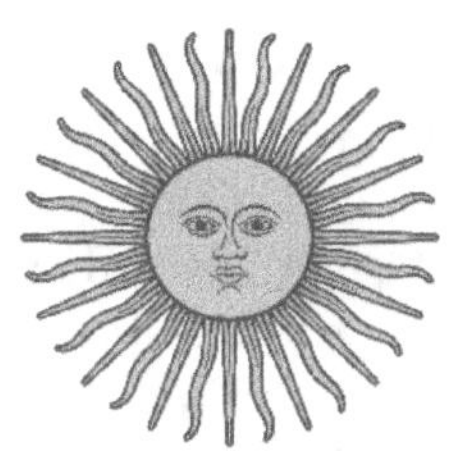

Conquering the Winter Blues

Over 60 Steps to Tackle

Seasonal Affective Disorder and Depression

By Ellie Hadsall

Conquering the Winter Blues

Over 60 Steps to Tackle
Seasonal Affective Disorder and Depression
By Ellie Hadsall
Photo by ChumelNZ, courtesy of Pixabay
Copyright © 2020 Ellie Hadsall

Table of Contents

What good is the warmth of summer,
without the cold of winter to give it sweetness.
- John Steinbeck

1

Addressing Winter Blues

*Love the person in the mirror. Everything they have
been through has been for your sake.*
- Ellie

Depression is debilitating any time of year, but when winter rolls around it can be overwhelming. But then, you already know that, or you wouldn't have chosen to read this book. I hope something included here can shift that for you, as it has for others.

Winter Blues is caused by lack of sunlight. Depression, on the other hand, has a multitude of causes. Thousands of people today experience depression. If you "think you might have it", you probably do. The suggestions in this book can help to alleviate either of these conditions.

Who am I to write this book? I'm not a doctor, research scientist, or psychologist. I'm an ordinary woman who has personally experienced depression and winter blues and survived. For over twenty-five years as a minister, I have mentored people facing these debilitating issues. This book will not present studies, research, or science to back up these ideas; you can find that online. What I offer here is lifestyle suggestions to apply during daily life. Guidelines in this book can offer help far beyond depression. These are guidelines for living a healthy, invigorating, and fulfilling life.

But let's just start with right now. Today. One step at a time.

I sank deeply into post-partum depression after giving birth to our first child. Several of the techniques offered in this book saved my sanity. (Details of these events are included in the "Author" chapter.) A few years later, we moved to a northern state, living where long, cold winters defined my world with sub-freezing temperatures, brooding grey clouds, and months of snowplowed streets lined with four-foot-high mounds of dirty, frozen snow.

I knew that I was fortunate to live in a warm, cozy house with a good husband, adorable toddler, and steaming cups of hot chocolate, but I desperately needed sunlight! The more I lamented lack of sunshine, the more it rattled my peace of mind. I finally remembered the practices I'd used to survive the post-partum months and so I began to pull myself out of the blue funk. I learned to meditate, which taught me how to control my thoughts instead of allowing them to control me. By intentionally applying a variety of specific practices, I recaptured my sense of self. Lesson was finally learned – again!

As a minister, I've now counseled a multitude of others who suffer winter blues or depression. At one time or another I've personally proven to myself that every suggestion in this book can help.

Over the years I've become convinced of a valuable lesson:

If someone applies even a few techniques diligently, consistently, and for at least three weeks, they can shift their outlook and begin liberating themselves from winter blues.

I seldom get hooked by cloudy and cold weather anymore, because most of these techniques have become my daily lifestyle. And I've learned that *if I diligently maintain my inner world of thought and self-reference as sunny, it radiates light onto my outer world circumstances.*

A few recommendations come from over thirty years of practicing Ayurveda, a healing and lifestyle system from ancient India. Similar practices are found in cultures across the globe. Most of these suggestions you may have heard of already and may be practicing. Here, I offer you a compilation for easy reference. But the key is to practice them on days when you don't feel like it. *Those are the days you need to be practicing them the most.*

So, what is Seasonal Affective Disorder (SAD)?

Also known as "Winter Blues" or "Cabin Fever", SAD is a depressed and withdrawn response to the short days of decreased sunlight, and long nights of late fall and winter seasons.

Decreased light affects sleep patterns and bio-rhythms. It affects four times as many women as men. Yet men and children can also suffer. SAD is severely debilitating to some and an inconvenience to others, but you don't have to merely tolerate it.

Natural, simple, and effective remedies are available. Unfortunately, *once you begin to suffer from winter blues you may lose interest in taking helpful action because of the depressed and unmotivated mood you experience.* It is necessary to make yourself commit to remedies. It's helpful to begin addressing it in October when the season begins, to catch it early. But anytime is the best time to begin.

This information is not intended to address severe or chronic depression.

This information focuses on lifestyle.

It does not include herbal, supplement, or medical advice.

If your depression has a cause deeper than SAD, or if winter intensifies an already-present depression, *please seek professional help.* Don't hole up alone and deepen your suffering. Do what is best for you, regardless of other people's well-intentioned and sometimes misplaced advice.

Counseling, anti-depressants, and knowing people who understand what you are experiencing, will help you through. If you've tried natural remedies that aren't working, pharmaceuticals can help stabilize you in order to experience the motivation or stamina to help yourself. Once you are more stable, you will find it easier to follow natural solutions. *Never judge yourself because you turn to medical help.* There is no right or wrong here. You have the right to take care of yourself in whatever way works for you.

You are valuable and worth the effort it takes to find your personal power!

How to Apply Lifestyle Suggestions

- Start out easy.

  Keep it simple. Making changes is challenging when you already feel overwhelmed by life. You may feel as if you don't have the energy to tackle your depression head-on. So, focus on only a few steps at a time.

- Apply choices with a regular routine.

  Follow them *consistently* in order to experience results. It is better to apply a few suggestions consistently than to try too many, get frustrated, and give up. In general, it is recommended to practice a new action for 21 days in order to change a life habit.

- Do additional practices as you have time, or on weekends.

- Not all practices work for everyone. If a suggestion doesn't work, after you have given it an honest try, move on to try another one.

Occasionally, you will see Sanskrit words written in *italics*. These practices are found in aforementioned ancient Vedic healing tradition known as Ayurveda, as well as in other traditions.

∾ *If you are focused on a self-realization or spiritual path, you may want to visit the "Self-Actualization and Spiritual" chapter first.* ∾

In summary...

To conquer Winter Blues and Depression, you can't wait for an outside force to magically shift your mood. You're going to have to take the lead in your life and blast through mental and physical obstacles. You'll need to do so with a *belief that you are worth it*, and a willingness to accept your own lightness-of-being.

This is why I chose a stag, whose antlers are adorned with joyful and abundant spring flowers, to adorn this book's cover.

A stag is an animal of power and vigor. As a totem, it represents the protector. Who, I ask, is your innate protector? It's *you*, at your strongest and best. The deer represents intuition and gentleness. It brings harmony, happiness, peace, and longevity.

With its antlers, the deer can push through forest obstacles. Antlers allow it to protect itself and those it loves from harm, and to prove its power with all that would challenge.

With colorful and healing flowers adorning its antlers, the stag carries along the light and joy of spring and summer as it moves through life, even into the occasional dark shadows of forest trees. And to top it all off, antlers represent a crown of achievement. Isn't it time to celebrate reconnecting with your own power?

Detailed information will be provided at the end of this book for the following:

- Emotion Vibration Chart

- Meditation

- Candle Gazing

- Self-Massage

- Breath of Fire

- Gayatri Mantra Chant

- Vedic Fire Blessing

- Make Space for Joy

Depression is not failure, weakness, wrong, stupid, embarrassment, or any of the multitude of emotions it ignites. Depression brings a sense of hopelessness, misery, isolation, timidity, fear, and exhaustion. None of these is the truth of who you really are.

Ready? Begin your journey to a better winter...

2

Light Therapy

Within you is the light of a thousand suns.
- Robert Adams

Lights! Lights! Lights!

Whether you suffer from SAD, temporary depression, or chronic depression, *Light Therapy is absolutely essential*. You need to replicate the sun's rays in any possible way.

Light is an environmental stimulus for regulating circadian cycles. When sunlight is lacking, the results can be mental or emotional discomfort. In severe cases, this can lead to SAD and depression.

Use Full Spectrum or Daylight bulbs and tubes.

Replace all light bulbs with full spectrum bulbs. Not all "Full Spectrum" or "Daylight" bulbs are produced the same. A full-spectrum/daylight bulb carries both visible and invisible color wavelengths of light colors, as does natural sunlight, and this light is distributed in equal proportions to natural light. Daylight lamps were created to simulate daylight for improved health to people who get limited or no exposure to the sun because of their profession, or who live in regions with short daylight hours. Some examples are residents of northern countries, astronauts in the space program, and personnel on Navy submarines.

Not all "full spectrum" bulbs on the market are distributed equally across the light spectrum, so educate yourself online before purchasing, and shop carefully.

LED bulbs can be a helpful substitute for the more expensive full-spectrum lights. While they don't emit the full spectrum, they are better than traditional incandescent or florescent bulbs.

Avoid fluorescent bulbs or spiral bulbs which are compact florescent bulbs (CFLs).

These fluorescent bulbs have negative effects on our circadian rhythms and are shown to cause body distress. If you work in a space with overhead florescent lights, respectfully request that they replace the bulbs with non-florescent, full-spectrum tubes. If they will not, consider paying for replacement bulbs yourself. Don't let your own health suffer because the company won't pay for something; do it on your own if possible. *Invest in yourself.*

For thirty years, my sister was a third-grade teacher in British Columbia, Canada. In winter, her town was bitterly cold and dry, with 17 to 18 days of −30 °C (−22 °F) temperatures and strong winds. She lamented how depressed the children became during the winter. She began to notice herself slipping into dark moods and a sense of hopelessness. I shipped her a box of full-spectrum bulbs for her home. She immediately took the box to the school to replace every light bulb in her classroom. Within only a few days, she noticed the children were calmer, more engaged, and happier. Another shipment of bulbs we sent were soon used to light her home. Overjoyed at the difference full spectrum light made, she approached the administration to request using them throughout the school, but unfortunately, they didn't want to invest. I've since learned that many schools in Canada and Scandinavian countries now utilize these as a regular practice.

<u>Author Reminder</u>: Some of the names, locations, and identifying characteristics have been changed to protect the privacy of those depicted.

Light Therapy Resources: Full Spectrum Solutions or Chromalux. Online searches offer numerous resources.

Light Box Therapy

During light therapy, you sit or work near a device called a light therapy box.

The "box" or special lamp gives off bright light that mimics natural outdoor light. Light therapy is thought to affect brain chemicals linked to mood and sleep, easing Seasonal Affective Disorder (SAD) symptoms. Using a light therapy box may also help with other types of depression, sleep disorders, and other conditions. Light therapy is also known as "bright light therapy" or "phototherapy". *It is estimated that 10,000 lux is needed for effective treatment of severe cases.*

It is recommended to use your light therapy lamp in the morning upon arising, imitating the natural rise of the sun. Using it at night can over-stimulate some people, leading to insomnia.

The key to success is consistency. Use it *every morning*. On days you feel good and are inclined to not use the light, commit to using it anyway. Missing even a few days can decrease the overall effectiveness.

Begin using light therapy in October and continue through winter.

Be aware that some "light boxes" provide light for other purposes that is focused toward only one area of the spectrum, such as blue or green, and thus are not full-spectrum. The resources I list below are authentic.

Resources: Verilux, Alaska Northern Lights, Light Therapy Products, Sun Box. Online searches offer numerous resources.

Take a small light therapy lamp to your job and set it in your work area.

Leave lights on around the house when you are home.

I realize this suggestion flies in the face of sustainable

living advice. While I champion a sustainable lifestyle, when it comes to personal depression, *light is paramount.* If you can't afford full-spectrum, use LEDs. Their power usage is minimal and far less than the incandescent bulbs available in the past.

During the winter, I turn on all upstairs lights when getting ready for the day, including our bedroom, hallway, and bathroom. This is to simulate sunshine radiating in all windows. Then I turn them off and move downstairs where I turn on all kitchen and dining room lights as I prepare and eat breakfast.

If the day is especially gloomy, I turn on all living room lights, too, so that my body senses as if the sunshine were bathing every room. I work in a home office, so keep all lights on in that room during a cloudy day. I open all curtains and shades in the entire house, so that as I move around, daylight enters each room. My windows offer an expanded view of the neighborhood that attracts my attention away from the darker house.

3

Attitude and Outlook

*It is easier to act your way into a new way
of thinking than it is to think your way into
a new way of acting.*
- Millard Fuller

Attitude and outlook determine how ready and willing you are to do what it takes to slay this dragon.

Are you ready to apply new ways of living in order to find relief?

You can't experience new results if you continue with the same old behavior and beliefs.

You have to care enough to get out of your current comfort zone to do things differently.

Embrace winter.

Winter will be what it will be. The key to survival is in finding its gifts.

People love to complain about the weather. The second greeting comment you often hear after, "How are you"? is a judgment on the weather. "It's too cold today," in wintertime, and "It's too hot today," in summer, as if this is an unusual occurrence worth noting. The more we complain about something, the more convinced we are that we are right. And the moment someone agrees with us, we are off and running with a long discussion of how we mutually suffer.

If you view winter as an enemy, you'll find constant confirmation that it's terrible. If you look for the positives in winter, you'll begin to see them more often. *What you focus on will increase.* Choose to not participate in mutual complaining and replace it with something positive and constructive that moves you away from a depression funk instead of deeper into it.

Raise your vibration.

Emotions carry a vibration. The higher the frequency of your energy or vibration, the lighter you feel in your body, emotions, and mind. If you raise your vibration, your emotions improve. A majority of the suggestions in this book will raise your vibration to a higher level, thus improving your daily experience. (*See "Emotion Vibration Chart" at end of book*)

Meditate.

My number one recommendation for any concern is to meditate. I've seen it change more people's lives than any other practice I know. Personally, I have continued a daily meditation practice for over forty years. Depression centers in the mind, and meditation brings mental clarity and self-compassion. Through consistent daily practice, meditation connects you with a higher, wiser, more assured Self. *(Details at end of book)*

Candle Gaze.

Candle Gazing is another proven method to calm anxiety and to nurture serenity, along with a multitude of other benefits. *(Details at end of book)*

Seek Counseling.

Depression is intensified anytime we feel trapped or stuck. Consider counseling to resolve personal issues. A willingness to seek counseling demonstrates courage! *(Also see "Counseling" chapter)*

Be a victor instead of a victim.

Buying into a victim mentality keeps you stuck and feeling heavy. Observe how you are identifying as a suffering, helpless victim of circumstances. Then take charge of your life and set about making necessary changes, one step at a time.

Monitor self-talk and delete negative thoughts.

At first, you may find your mind is filled with constant negative talk.

"Today is not going to be a good day."

"I'm constantly depressed."

"It's cloudy; the sun isn't shining – again!"

The moment you become aware of such thoughts, stop them. Simply shut off the attention and the thought will lose power. Consistently shut off the attention, and the power will fizzle out.

Avoid judging the daily weather and outside circumstances.

Instead of judging a winter day as good or bad, look at it "as it is". When you face the facts and allow that they are "as they are", you no longer have to expend mental effort by resisting anything you judge as "wrong".

Weather is. Winter is. Cold is. Cloudy is.

Release judging it and release the resistance. If you can't change something, accept it and set about finding a way to improve on it. This opens up room for possibilities.

When other's comment negatively about the weather, a simple response such as, "Yes, it is cloudy, and I intend to make the best of it," and then changing the subject, will help move the conversation forward.

Focus on the positive.

At work and home, commit to looking for and focusing on the many positives that *are* in your life.

Life brings challenges and everyone has unwanted experiences, yet focusing on the positive is proven to change one's outlook. Discipline your thoughts to move away from the darkness that cloudy days bring. Choose a positive thought, image, mantra, prayer, affirmation, or even a positive word and immediately transfer your thoughts from the negative over to your preferred positive focus.

One cloudy winter, to test this theory, I decided to choose something ridiculous to focus on. I decided nothing could be sillier than "ice cream", so I set it as my distraction focus. Whenever I started to feel panicky about the clouds, I immediately envisioned an ice cream cone stacked with tasty flavors. As my mind created various flavors with their accompanying color and scent, my mind became engaged, and I forgot to be panicky.

I learned to distract myself from mental misery. This helped liberate me from depression. A woman I know moves her attention toward imagining her dream home. A basketball player refocuses attention to mentally shooting hoops. Over the years, I've consistently used this technique to transfer my thoughts from negative to positive. I've substituted negative thoughts with affirmations, visualizations, or singing a song. There are no rules here. When you need a "thought" lifeline, grab whatever you can to rescue yourself from going down that mental rabbit hole. It if works for you, it's a success!

Whatever diverting focus you choose, be sure it's positive and optimistic!

Keep a positives/gratitude journal.

Every night prior to bed, write down at least three positives from your day. It can include what someone did for you, what you accomplished, or something fun or interesting that you heard. Do not go to sleep until you write down at least three things from that day that you can appreciate. This encourages you to intentionally create positive experiences so you will have an entry for the evening journal. Further, it primes your mind to seek out positives as the day progresses.

When facing a series of difficult circumstances, I began a positive journal. One evening, I could not think of anything positive that had happened that day. I tried to go to bed with no journal entries, but I couldn't sleep. I made myself get out of bed to make three positive things happen. I opened the fridge to get a snack and noticed it was too dirty, so spent the next hour tossing left-overs and cleaning. I sent a thank-you email to a friend. Then I entered our two daughters' rooms to lean over and gratefully kiss each on the forehead. Satisfied, and feeling good about my day, I went to sleep happy.

Express appreciation and gratitude daily.

When I'm feeling down, I push myself to be kind to everyone, including total strangers. It never fails to pull me out of a blue funk.

Feeling tired and overextended, I maneuvered my way through the grocery aisles, finishing up with a trip down the hair care aisle for shampoo. Reaching across a woman who was stocking the shelves, I secured my choice and then paused.

"Thanks for stocking the shelves. It's one of those niceties we take for granted but never give thought

to the people behind the scenes who do the work."

She turned with a smile. "Thank you! I've worked here for over thirty years and few people ever notice the work we do."

This led to a conversation about her finding the job, working while raising two children, going through a divorce, and now nearing retirement. "These people I work with have been my family. They've helped me through a lot of problem years!"

During our conversation, she had tears in her eyes. Finally, she said, "Today has been a difficult day for me. One of my sons just told me he has cancer. I'm thankful you stopped to talk. I think you were supposed to, don't you?"

We hugged, she picked up a bottle of conditioner to place on the shelf and I checked out. No longer tired, no longer overwhelmed, I now felt the joy of sharing a compassionate moment with a fellow human.

Smile

Smile, whether you "feel" like it or not, including when you are alone. Studies indicate that smiling - even when you have to make yourself do so - activates neuropeptides in your brain that control stress. It also releases dopamine, endorphins and serotonin which are associated with lowering anxiety and increasing happiness. Serotonin is often the chemical that anti-depressant medications regulate. You begin to feel happier and more relaxed. An added benefit is that others perceive and respond to you in a more positive way, which helps lift your mood.

Laugh!

Watch funny movies, attend comedy clubs, join or start a laughter group.

Avoid dark, demeaning comedy or cutting sarcasm, which lower your vibration. Happy, hearty laughter produces endorphins, strengthens the diaphragm, increases blood flow, and encourages deep breathing which revitalizes the body.

Amanda was experiencing agoraphobia. A series of traumatic events had turned this outgoing woman into a recluse who barely had courage to take her dogs for a walk. At her low point, she arranged for groceries to be delivered in order to avoid facing crowds. Desperate for help, and having heard that humor heals, she forced herself to go to the library to check out comedy videos. Returning those movies, she checked out more. What began as slight smiles became chuckles, evolving into loud hoots. "A strong laugh felt fresh, exhilarating, and totally liberating!" Along with the laughter, Amanda regained a positive outlook, confidence, and hope. She now offers seminars on laughter yoga and is once again actively involved in her community. Today, her agoraphobia is only a memory.

Help yourself out by giving a few of these ideas a try!

4

Counseling

When we are no longer able to change a situation,
we are challenged to change ourselves.
– Victor Frankl

You are the master of your life.

Being master of our life means being self-accountable.

It requires seeing things for the truth of what they are and finding personal solutions.

No one else can heal you. It is up to you to heal yourself. If you don't know how, counseling offers support with a wide variety of options.

Wounded emotions, poor environmental conditions, fatigue, undue stress, and poor nutrition affect our mood and state of mind, as do chemical and hormonal imbalances. Seeking someone else to save us, looking for the perfect mate, promiscuity, drugs, alcohol, shopping, gambling, over-exercising, refusing to eat or overeating, gambling, self-harming, extreme isolation, and over-working are rampant indicators of people desperately seeking refuge from trauma. Depression is a common denominator in all of these.

Deep within the subconscious, we hold beliefs and perceptions that control the majority of our decisions. We can notice life unraveling and want to stop it, yet we are deeply fearful of confronting the traumas that influence our current reality.

Unfortunately, counseling is still misunderstood by many to be reserved for crazy people, or weaklings that can't tough life out. Nothing could be further from the truth. Counseling takes courage. It invites you to face the fear, pain, and anger of past trauma which formed your current situation of depression, addiction, or avoidance. With counseling, we discover misperceptions and habits that keep us stuck. We learn proven processes to resolve them.

Past trauma that is anchored in our body can be released so we can live in the present without being bound up by old wounds. Post-traumatic stress is labeled as a "disorder" (PTSD), but I don't perceive it as a disorder at all. It is a normal survival mechanism that our subconscious uses to keep us safe – but in today's world it keeps us stuck. New methods are being discovered daily that help heal the past.

> *Expand your healing beyond finger pointing.*
> *The best healing tool is a willingness to be*
> *self-accountable with your life.*

Types of Counselors and Therapists

A psychiatrist is a physician (MD) who, after medical school, has completed additional training in psychiatry.

An advanced practice or psychiatric/mental health nurse practitioner (ARNP or PMHNP) is a nurse who has completed a nursing degree and additional training in psychiatry.

A psychologist has received a PhD in psychology and can carry the title of "doctor". Psychologists are able to administer a variety of tests.

Master's level clinicians include social workers (LICSW, MSW), mental health counselors (LMHC), licensed professional counselors (LPC), and marriage and family therapists (LMFT).

All of the above have varying levels of medical privileges and ability to prescribe medicines.

Types of Healing Modalities

I include here a brief glimpse of only a few of the possible therapy modalities. No one method holds all the answers for everyone. Often people benefit by eventually utilizing more than one. If you experience deep-seated trauma that causes you to act irrationally at times, don't berate yourself. Instead, seek a psychologist or psychotherapist who can offer medications if needed to help you through the rough healing crises until you are more stable.

Healing the Inner Child

Inner child therapy is part of most healing modalities. It guides us to heal traumatic childhood events. We can review them from a safe perspective as an adult, release the emotional trauma from the subconscious, and recapture our power.

The first six to seven years of life form our childhood reality. During those years, our reasoning ability has not yet flowered. We record what we experience as reality, but it is being viewed with a naïve, innocent, immature, and inexperienced perception.

As we witness our environment, we decide how to cope and survive in this physical reality. We form our "shoulds" and "musts". We learn what is safe and what we need to avoid. If our surroundings and family life is healthy and empowering, we develop with strong role models. If our situation is dysfunctional, traumatic, or confusing, we develop survival skills that hinder healthy and empowering relationships when we apply them to our reasoning and social interaction as we reach school years and in later adult life.

As a child, learning to placate an angry mother will condition us to eventually placate an angry spouse. Sexual abuse from an older male cousin will condition us to distrust males. Subsequent adult behavior choices, that are based on childhood subconscious conditionings, will elicit dysfunctional responses from others and thus "prove" our false perceptions to be true.

These subconscious, conditioned habits and beliefs are a program that runs our adult life more than ninety percent of the time. Yet part of us senses something is wrong. An inner struggle ensues. Is it any wonder that we feel depressed, trapped, hopeless, and exhausted?

Many of the following modalities access these childhood patterns as part of the healing process. My explanations are basic. I recommend going online to do further reading on each modality.

Emotional Memory Therapy (EMT)

Emotional Memory Therapy adapts, alters, and improves memory of emotional events or stimuli. When the client recognizes the connection between memory and current emotional stimuli, they can learn techniques to effectively manage it. Outdated and ineffective survival patterns that drive our current behavior are resolved through use of new and proven tools and skills. EMT may include a variety of approaches.

Emotional Freedom Technique (EFT)

EFT is also known as "tapping", "meridian tapping" or "acupressure tapping". The client taps on specific points on the body as they process through a verbal or visual process. Points of tapping connect with the body's energy in a way that helps relieve negative symptoms. EFT is frequently integrated with other modalities.

Eye Movement Desensitization and Reprocessing (EMDR)

Studies indicate that EMDR brings benefits that used to take years to achieve. It is based on a concept that the mind can heal itself, much as the rest of the body can heal itself after an injury. Distressing thoughts and emotions are blended with new positive thoughts and emotions. Energy blocks from emotional wounds dissipate and issues are resolved through healing movements.

Gestalt Therapy

The word "gestalt" means "whole". With gestalt, one perceives the wholeness of a situation, with a new ability to perceive it from all angles. A gestalt therapist guides you to review a distressing or confusing past experience in order to gain new awareness and insight.

The gestalt focus is to experience the feelings rather than to talk about or analyze them logically. This therapy may include working with role-play, confrontation, or dreams.

Personally, I utilize gestalt in everyday life in order to assess past and present situations. Once the truth of the situation is understood from all angles, I am better suited to address the circumstances in a mature, confident, and compassionate manner.

Therapeutic Trembling

Trembling and shaking are natural reactions to trauma. Social pressure to "keep your cool" requires us to block these natural responses. Shaking helps release the over-stimulation of the "fight or flight" response.

When we stifle this natural response, that tension is then trapped in our bodies, causing undue stresses, and blocking blood flow and nerve impulses.

With Therapeutic Trembling, we are guided to tremble, shake, and release stored stress so our body can once more function with wholeness.

When applied in refugee camps with children and adults who have fled horrific events, Therapeutic Trembling has proven a powerful healing modality.

Childhood Regression Hypnotherapy

Through use of a mild form of hypnosis, a therapist helps the client to access the subconscious mind where memories are stored. The client discovers hidden trauma, obstacles, and conflicts that influence their current life.

By recognizing the original cause of current confusion or suffering, a new understanding emerges that can resolve issues and bring a newfound sense of wholeness. Surprisingly, many revealed memories are not necessarily traumatic in themselves, but instead offer new insights.

Life Regression Hypnotherapy

Often known as "Past Life Regression Therapy", this modality emerged from the earlier practice of Childhood Regression Therapy. During regression sessions, occasional clients reported memory of events in another life. With research, many of these reports were eventually authenticated when details of the client's memory matched up with real life documentation.

As with Childhood Regression, discovering the original cause of one's current distress, in a different lifetime, can offer insight, bring resolution, and expand understanding. Many spiritual traditions, as well as testimony from highly respected people, have suggested we live multiple lifetimes.

Quantum physics is revealing the possibility of parallel worlds. Leading science suggests alternate lives may be simultaneous rather than linear. This is a leading-edge modality. I have personally seen it transform people's lives.

Resource: "Alternate Lives of Ruthye", by Ruthye Preston, shares her personal revelation of over thirty alternate lifetimes and how they influence her current life and self-evolution. Available on Amazon.

A Special Note about Nature's Pharmaceuticals

Psilocybin Therapy (from certain varieties of hallucinogenic mushrooms), Cannabis (as medical marijuana), and CBD (a variety of compounds derived from cannabis) are all being studied for their ability to decrease depression.

The FDA has designated Psilocybin Therapy as "breakthrough therapy", a designation that allows it to be accelerated through their drug development and review trials, as treatment for major depressive disorder. While not legal in some places, these natural remedies are increasingly considered serious methods of treatment. You can find research online. Stay tuned!

Example of Combined Modalities

Nikki hated her job. Every morning she dreaded going to work and spent her weekends holed up in her home, feeling depressed and hopeless. In February, after a long winter, she began considering suicide. Nothing in her life was working. She had a good job that afforded her to own a home, but she was constantly anxious and never felt safe. She had a driving desire to please other people, especially men. She felt her current male manager demeaned her work and she daily considered finding another job that was better - a pattern she had followed through three previous jobs. Desperate, she sought counseling.

Nikki's counselor began with a childhood regression session. Nikki, her older brother Robbie, and little sister were raised by a financially strapped single mother. Her father was a financially successful man, prominent in the community, who neglected to pay child support. When the therapist led Nikki into her session, Nikki remembered a day when she was nine, standing in her bedroom as her big brother, Robbie, taunted her.

Nikki had suggested to him that she was going to ask their paternal grandmother to help them. Robbie laughed and yelled at her, "You are so stupid! Why would she listen to you? You're such a loser!" He continued ranting at her about how she wore her hair, her poor grades at school, how he hated living in a house with all girls, and how he couldn't wait to get out of there to make his own money, like their father.

She had run crying out into the back yard to hide behind the shed where she went when she wanted to be alone. She remembered picking up a stick and stabbing it in the ground as she decided she hated men who had power and money. She was going to avoid them when she grew up so she would be safe.

Bringing the session to an end, Nikki's therapist took her through a process to nurture her nine-year-old-self and then led her out of the memory and back into the present moment.

On the next visit, the therapist led Nikki through a gestalt session where Nikki role-played an imaginary conversation with her brother. During that session, she realized that Robbie was carrying deep scars from his father's rejection. He was scared and lonely. He struck out at her and everyone around him as a way to protect himself from the pain of being seen as weak and useless. As an adult, Robbie had become a driven man, successful in his own right, and he was now on his third marriage. Nikki realized her decision to not trust strong men had subconsciously been transferred to every male manager she had worked for.

With her therapist's guidance, Nikki learned to see herself as a capable woman. She learned how to be more assertive at work. With her new perspective and understanding, she realized that her current manager had been supportive of her, but her own sensitivity had consistently misinterpreted what she was experiencing at work. Today, Nikki supervises a department in that corporation and is dating an attorney who respects her and champions her abilities. No longer encumbered by her childhood trauma, she is free to live fully in the present.

Don't stumble over something behind you.
\- Seneca

5

Nutrition

Our food should be our medicine,
and our medicine should be our food.
- Hippocrates

Drink at least 32 ounces of water daily.

Fill a quart glass bottle with room-temperature water and sip on it throughout the day. When craving sweets or caffeine, drink water first which may allow your craving to dissipate. Note: recommendations on required water amounts vary widely and depend on your personal body and lifestyle needs. 32 ounces is a general standard.

Limit carbohydrates. Eat lean protein and leafy greens.

Carbohydrates make people feel heavy, sluggish, are high in calories, and hold little nutritional value.

Eat warm, moist, well-cooked foods such as soups and sautés.

In cold weather, avoid foods that are raw and cold. According to Ayurveda, fall and winter cold temperatures and wind stir up fear and anxiety. Depression is supported by subconscious beliefs and feelings of anxiety, abandonment, unworthiness, and loneliness. Warm, cooked foods offer nurturing, comfort, and are easier to digest in cold climates.

Avoid or limit sugar.

Sugar highs that seem to lift your spirits will end in a depressive crash. Sugar creates an unnatural energy boost which causes your body to decrease its glucose output. When the sugar boost wears off, and your body is no longer producing necessary glucose, you crash until your body has time to increase its glucose output. A crash brings exhaustion and depression.

I know I am the only one on planet Earth to have done this - but I used to depend upon cookies or snacks to lift my mood. I'd indulge, but a few hours later I felt lethargic, even exhausted. I worked in a two-story office building and by afternoon I'd feel as if I could barely make it up the stairs. When I cut back on sugar, my energy became steady and dependable. I no longer had to "grab something sweet, or have a cup of coffee, or a coke" to boost my energy. I still love cookies, and sugar in my coffee! But when I keep it to a minimum, steady energy carries me through the day with no slumps.

Avoid or minimize alcohol.

Alcohol is a depressant, and it also affects glucose because of its high sugar content. A glass of wine can relax you, yet eventually leads to a sugar crash.

Avoid excessive caffeine.

After the initial energy boost caffeine brings, it is followed by an energy crash, similar to sugar.

Quality *dark* chocolate is a mood lifter.

*I am a woman of many moods
and they all require chocolate.*

Studies show that dark chocolate, of at least 70% cocoa, can lift a mood. Just don't overdo, because it does contain caffeine.

When serving as education director of a school, I sought to keep an open heart with each student and staff member that approached me. I frequently worked ten-hour days and often helped students on weekends. By mid-afternoon, my energy lagged and I desperately craved a nap.

I'll bet you can identify with that! I discovered that if I savored a small piece of dark chocolate, I felt love well up within my heart, and I was back on track. Rumor has it that some yogis eat a bit of chocolate before meditating to open their heart and keep them alert. That's one rumor I've decided to believe!

6

Self Care

*How we care for ourselves gives our brain messages
that shape our self-worth, so we must care
for ourselves in every way, every day.*
- Sam Owen

Create a regular morning routine.

Schedule at least a few regular morning practices as a routine. You'll feel "on top of the day" instead of under a cloud. Prepare the night before, set your alarm, and get up to do them regardless of whether you feel like it. Consistency is essential. Do at least 20-30 minutes of physical activity, followed by meditation and/or prayer to focus on positive aspects before moving on with your day.

Bathe or shower every morning.

Water provides negative ions which promote serotonin in the brain, which is a mood lifter. Even if you don't feel dirty, at least have a quick rinse. If water is limited, freshen up with water in the morning to get a lift.

Bathe or shower with full appreciation to your body, hair, and skin – *as it is now.*

Release judgment of your body. The human body comes in all shapes and sizes. It is an amazing gift that self-heals, adjusts to our needs, and sustains us through all circumstances. Think of your body as a companion that is there for you regardless of the circumstances, and then set about taking care of it as best you can.

Give a Self-Massage.

At least once a week, give yourself a full body self-massage with warm oil. Sit 10-15 minutes. Shower off. *(Details at end of book)*

Get a professional massage.

A massage stimulates your circulation, releases stress from muscles, and encourages body relaxation. If you live in an area with a massage school, they may offer discounted massages from their students.

Use Essential Oils.

Place a drop of essential oil on pulse points and soles of your feet or mix it into lotion.

Use oil drops in a room diffuser, or on a lamp bulb ring.

Use essential oil in morning and throughout the day as needed.

The following oils are a few suggestions that are mood lifting, inspirational, and anti-depressant.

- Bergamot (motivating, uplifting, productive)
- Lemon, orange, orange blossom, grapefruit, ginger (energizing, uplifting)
- Clary sage (antidepressant)
- Lavender, Ylang Ylang (calming, soothing)
- More suggestions can be found online

Wear color shades of yellow, orange, and tangerine (sun colors).

Stick with light, bright, or pastel colors. Avoid dark, dull colors such as grey, brown, and black. If you wear them, accessorize with colorful neckties, sweaters, scarves, or jewelry to add vitality.

Dress warmly in cold or windy weather.

Keep your head, neck, and extremities warm. If you chill easily, wear turtle-necks or wrap a scarf around your neck. Wear a warm cap and muffler when going outdoors. According to the science of Ayurveda, wind and cold can stir up fear, anxiety, and insecurity.

Get regular health care evaluations.

Winter Blues or depression can indicate hormonal or other physical imbalances that are aggravated by long, dark winter days. Hormonal imbalances frequently cause distress in women. My early episode of postpartum blues was caused by hormonal imbalances as my body readjusted from the hormonal changes necessary for the pregnancy. Peri and post-menopausal mood swings and depression can be equally distressing. Men are also affected by hormone imbalances which can contribute to depression and lethargy. Your doctor or health care practitioner can assess your situation and offer solutions if needed.

7

Electronics

*All this modern technology just makes people
try to do everything at once.*
- Bill Watterson

About Electronics...

Electrical equipment and electronic devices emit
Electromagnetic Fields (EMFs). This includes cell
phones, laptops, computers, wireless game systems,
smart televisions, and any technology utilizing 4G,
5G and WIFI. Studies indicate even this low level of
radiation can cause negative effects on humans.
EMFs are shown to disrupt our sleep cycles and nerve
networks.

*I used to carry a cell phone in my left trouser pocket
until the day I lost all feeling and movement in my
left leg. The culprit was my cell phone. I am thankful
I discovered the cause before I experienced
permanent damage. I no longer carry it on me but
place it on a table in the room where I am working.
When I need to keep it with me, I carry it in a small*

bag slung over my shoulder.

Avoid electronics first thing in the morning.

Electronic emissions inhibit the nervous system. That's a negative impact on someone who is already experiencing depression. Wait until you finish your morning routine of exercise, meditation, and showering before you leap on the electronic bandwagon. Then I highly recommend starting the day with a positive podcast, or positive social media page that is encouraging.

Don't get on electronics within an hour of bedtime.

Listening to calming music or brain-balancing tones is an exception but set your player or phone on a timer so you don't sleep with electronic devices near your body for the full night. As stated above, electronics disrupt our sleep cycle. Lack of sleep exacerbates depression.

Place electronics away from your bed.

Place your phone, tablet, and computer at least four feet away from your bed when you sleep.

Wear computer glasses.

Computer glasses are engineered to eliminate digital eye strain and block blue light that radiates from electronic devices, including smartphones, tablets, LCD TVs, and computers. This blue light stimulates the circadian rhythm which controls your biological clock. It can keep you awake and disrupt sleep. Some people report having dry eyes, slight headaches, body aches, and a general sense of body discomfort when using electronic devices for extended periods of time. My computer glasses allow me to write for long hours at my computer without suffering dry eyes and aches that I used to experience.

Ground yourself. Practice Earthing.

Walking barefoot on the dirt, grass, sand, or in water will connect your body with negative electrons. These negative electrons are absorbed by the body to neutralize the effects of invisible electromagnetic fields (EMFs) that surround us. They also neutralize free radicals.

Grounding appears to improve sleep, help address pain, reduce cortisol, reduce inflammation, and offers many additional benefits. There are numerous reports of depression being alleviated by consistent, daily grounding. It's not feasible to walk barefoot through the winter snow or on icy sidewalks, but there are a multitude of grounding devices available including shoes, sheets, and mats.

Resource: www.earthing.com

8

Exercise and Nature

*My grandmother started walking five miles a day
when she was sixty. She's ninety-seven now,
and we don't know where the heck she is.*
- Ellen DeGeneres

Breathe!

When depressed or anxious, we often forget to breathe deeply, or we hold our breath. Lack of fresh oxygen contributes to low energy and lethargy.

- *Breath of Fire* builds energy and stamina.

  By increasing the oxygen in your blood, your organs function better and your spirits are lifted. *(Breath of Fire details are at end of book.)*

- *Two-to-One Breath* calms anxiety and soothes depression.

  For each breath, exhale twice as long as the inhalation. For example, if you count to 3 while inhaling, count to 6 while exhaling. When stressed, we tend to breathe rapidly, hold our breath, or to exhale quickly. This signals our body to accelerate heart rate, raise blood pressure, and increasing tension in our muscles. By exhaling thoroughly with Two-One Breath, we slow the heart rate, lower blood pressure, and relax. Benefits of this are that it can be performed anywhere at any time. I practice it throughout the day to keep my energy balanced and steady.

Spend time with Mother Nature.

Take daily walks. Consider walking as part of your morning routine. Bundle up and go for a walk around the block or in a park, hike in the woods, or sit by a river or stream. What do you see, hear, smell, touch? Notice nature – trees, animals, tracks in snow, smell the freshness. Sun energy permeates nature even on a cloudy day. Outdoor morning energy is expansive.

When the sun is out, stand facing it and gaze near it (not directly) so light enters your eyes and thus the pineal gland which regulates glands and moods. Or sit in the sun with closed eyes and allow it to shine on your eyelids and forehead (where it enters the pineal gland). Do this outdoors if you can; or do it indoors near a window where sunshine enters.

Exercise actively at least three times a week.

Join a yoga, tai chi, or exercise class. There may be a yoga class in your area that focuses on Yoga for Depression. If not, ask a local yoga instructor for suggestions on yoga postures to address depression. You can also exercise at home.

I had knee issues and my physical therapist recommended special exercises and a stationary bike. We purchased a bike on sale and set it up in our basement. (You can often buy good used workout equipment because so many people buy them but never use them.) My legs have regained strength and are now stronger than they were twenty years ago. When exercising, I watch movies or listen to positive podcasts or music which engages my mind, so I don't become bored.

Roll!

Remember rolling across the grass or down a hill when you were a kid? Daily, clear back the furniture, get down on the floor, and roll back and forth across the room for at least two minutes. Rolling has been shown to open the heart, improve circulation, massage fascia and muscles, stimulate new neural pathways, release endorphins, and most of all, to spark joy! You can't help but feel silly as you roll. Hopefully, you'll feel like laughing which brings its own benefits. If you don't remember how to roll, you can find instructions online.

Play in the snow.

Bundle up so you can enjoy the cold. It's easy to find affordable high-tech clothing to keep warm. If finances are a problem, you can find plenty of options at your local thrift store. Before wearing used clothing, wash them first to remove the residual energy vibration of the previous owner.

Build a creative snowperson. Create snow sculptures. Make snow ice cream. Pour water over a yard of snow and play hockey with cups and a broom. Pour a stream of honey into shapes on the snow and snack on the frozen honey. Ice skate. Sled. Ski. Snowboard. Trek with snowshoes.

Ground yourself. Practice Earthing.

Grounding helps counteract the effects of EMFs. See the previous chapter on "Electronics" for details on Earthing.

Join the YMCA or a Fitness Club.

Working out is not about having a perfect body.
It's about creating a body you feel good in.
- Ellie

Joining an organization can keep you motivated. Research first to find one where you feel welcome and encouraged. You don't have to have a svelte or buff body, or cool clothes to work out.

YMCA offers affordable opportunities. Swim, learn a sport, work out, and be around other people. Even if you do not engage in conversation, the interaction helps stimulate your mind.

I had never worked out on equipment at a sports club but when a small local gym opened up a mile from our home, it seemed like a good idea. I kept putting it off, dreading being in a room full of people who looked like the perfect people in gym commercials. This was ridiculous because I practiced yoga daily and jogged a mile every morning, but vanity can put blinders on a person. So can depression.

Finally gathering courage, I went for my first visit. Working out at the gym with me that first day were real people - a man recovering from recent heart surgery, a high school football player, two women in their twenties, a mid-thirties woman trying to lose weight, and a seventy-year-old man with severe arthritis. I began regular work outs and chalked the experience up to one more life lesson I needed to learn.

Don't let your fear of other people's opinions keep you from taking care of yourself. Take charge of your own life and do what you need to do to feel good in your own skin.

9

Pets

*Until one has loved an animal,
a part of one's soul remains unawakened.*
- Anatole France

Pets offer companionship and comfort.

Whether you are a cat, dog, bird, fish, or reptile person, having one or more pets in your home brings an extra measure of vitality and silliness. Caring for them brings a sense of responsibility and self-worth.

Birds can be great companions.

Parrots and other birds that can mimic words and sounds can be engaging.

A friend of mine has a rescued grey parrot that greets her when she returns home, wishes her goodbye, and teases her. One of his favorite games is "Knock Knock". He makes a knocking sound until she responds, "Who's there?" Or, alternately, she knocks on wood, and he responds, "Who's there?" At times he breaks into raucous laughter until she can't help but respond in kind. Another friend has a bird that makes little soothing chirping noises when she is sad.

Dogs bring comfort.

There is a reason that dogs are the number one service animal. Dogs *care.*

Walking a dog takes you out into the world where you meet other people and momentarily get out of your own funk.

A few dog breeds that offer emotional support include King Charles Spaniel, Border Collie, Golden Retrievers, Greyhounds, Whippets, Pugs, Labrador Retriever, Poodle, and Yorkshire Terrier. These breeds tend to bond with their owner and enjoy their company without being too demanding.

Of course, dog personalities vary greatly. If you prefer rescue dogs as I do, the organization housing them often has a history of their personality.

Randy and his wife had a mid-sized, black, long-haired, mixed-breed rescue dog named Betty Boop. Betty had attached herself to Randy's wife and rarely interacted with him. Then Randy had a stroke and although he recovered well, he became depressed and spent most of his time in a chair watching television.

From the moment Randy returned home from the hospital, Betty Boop began following him everywhere. She slept by his side of the bed at night and at his feet when he sat in his chair. She insisted on licking his face occasionally and although formerly that would have irritated him, now it made him laugh. She harassed him when she wanted to go outside, forcing him to get up and take her out. As Randy healed and became more active, his confidence returned. By this time, he and Betty Boop had become best friends. Randy tells everyone that Betty rescued him. "I felt weak and useless, but she insisted I get back into the world."

Cats are independent and entertaining.

Nothing breaks me into laughter quicker than when our cat madly tears around the room, attacking table legs, and then dropping down serenely as if she just awoke from a nap. Her shenanigans are delightful and when she curls up to purr on my lap, her purring brings calm and peace.

Types of cat breeds that offer emotional support include American Shorthair (the most common cat), Main Coon, Ragdoll, Persian, Manx, and Sphynx. As with dogs, cat personalities vary greatly. If you prefer rescue cats as I do, the organization housing them often has a history of their personality.

A Word of Caution...

Pets require attention, maintenance, expensive veterinary care, and tons of love. It's essential to provide an environment where they feel free and loved. If you already lack energy for daily living, a pet will add additional havoc in your life. On the other hand, they also require you to get up, get out, and get into living. Think this through carefully.

If you love animals but aren't sure if that is the right thing for you to do, consider fostering an animal for a while to see if a pet is a good fit for you right now. And never give a pet to someone else, thinking you are doing a good deed. Check first to see if they want the responsibility.

10

Social

Reading something inspirational is not the same as doing something inspirational. Until you take action, inspiration is only a charming concept.
- Ellie

Holidays can contribute to depression.

Do you dread holidays? Maybe your family isn't one you'd choose. Perhaps you have no one to share it with, so the loneliness becomes overpowering. For many, holidays require attending boring or anxiety-filled parties and events.

It's your life and you have the right to live it the highest and best way you can. You have a right to not participate with any event that feels unreasonably demanding, demeaning, heavy, or oppressive.

If gatherings are a chore, maybe it's time to say "no". If family is not respectful to you now, politely declining a holiday gathering is not going to change their already-unpleasant attitude, and it will help you regain personal control over your life.

When attending any gathering with reluctance, instead of resisting the situation, try focusing on raising other people's spirits. Look around the room for someone who is alone or sad. Intentionally seek to help them feel better. This is a sure way to raise your own spirits, too.

As I was getting my hair cut before a Christmas party, my hairdresser bemoaned his family's Christmas requirements.

"I have to buy gifts for my parents, two sisters, their husbands, and their five kids. I don't even know what to get anyone, and I usually don't like what they give me. They have no idea who I really am. And I have to buy an expensive airplane ticket to fly across country, and face endless delays at airports. One of my sisters fights with Mom the whole time while the other sister drinks herself into oblivion. My brothers-in-law constantly talk about sports which bores me to death. I dread the holiday! I'd rather just visit my parents during the summer when it's quieter and we can have real conversations."

When I suggested he respectfully explain that his finances were insufficient to buy gifts or a ticket, and to arrange to visit in the summer as he preferred, he exclaimed, "No way! My family would never forgive me!"

Life's too precious to waste being in miserable company that only serves to deepen your depression. You can love family yet still prefer to spend time with your chosen family of friends.

Choose to be a victor, not a victim.

Invite others to your home on depressing holidays.

Who else do you know who is alone? Who else would appreciate companionship and a sense of feeling welcomed? Invite them to your home for a few hours, or go to a restaurant or movie together.

Give yourself permission to revel in the joy of spending a holiday alone.

When alone on a holiday, instead of regretting not being with others, plan a special day for yourself. Watch movies, take a long nap, work on a hobby. If you are an introvert, enjoy your time alone without feeling you "should" be out with other people.

Create your own reason for a gathering.

Introduce enjoyable ideas such as creating vision boards, cooking new recipes together, or everyone scattering around to read a good book while drinking hot toddies and munching on goodies.

Host a potluck.

For variety, invite everyone to bring a dish from their cultural tradition. Purchased food is approvable – not everyone likes to cook.

Hold a decadent dessert gathering where everyone brings their favorite treat. Choose a theme such as tantalizing chocolate desserts or scrumptious cakes.

Consider hosting a "Loaf of bread, jug of wine, and thou" party. Don't forget to add chocolate to the menu!

On a diet? Invite everyone to bring their favorite healthy dish.

Watch a sports game or enjoy an inspiring or funny movie.

Volunteer to help others.

Focus on helping others who are less fortunate. Contact a local church or organization to learn of families in need, and take them groceries, clothing, or other supplies. Any time we express kindness to others, we open our hearts and release endorphins. Bake meals, freeze in containers, and take to a shut in. The list of opportunities is endless!

Visit coffee or tea shops.

Chat with other patrons or simply people-watch.

Working on your computer at a local hangout can assuage loneliness and isolation.

Dance with friends, groups, or take dance lessons.

Join Meetup or Facebook groups on subjects of interest, or on totally new ideas.

Connect with others who experience SAD for reassurance and mutual support.

The worst thing to do is to isolate yourself. Share your concerns with others who can understand, while simultaneously encouraging each other toward solutions. Gather with other people!

Jenny was an introvert who suffered SAD. Out of desperation, she started a Meetup group for SAD people who considered themselves to be introverts.

The response was overwhelming, and she almost canceled out of fear. Forcing herself to continue, she invited them to meet in her home. Three women and one man attended and together they discussed their sense of isolation, dislike of social events, and shared ideas on how to deal with their depression. They decided to each keep track of what triggered their depression, to write down all of the good things in their lives, and to share these with each other at the next meeting.

The group has grown to an average of eight people who meet monthly. At each meeting, they agree to a focus for the next month and make a commitment to report back to the group. Jenny reports that her confidence has grown, she is more at ease at social events, and her former sense of isolation is dissolving.

When with others, agree to not complain, gossip, or whine.

It is healing to share concerns with others, knowing they understand and empathize with our situation. Then, it's time to move on. Constant negativity reinforces the blues when two or more people dwell on wrongs and reinforce each other's depression.

11

Environment

Decorate your home. It gives the illusion that
your life is more interesting than it really is.
- Charles M. Schulz

Redecorate your home in comforting, enlivening colors.

Once you redecorate your home, life actually does become more interesting. A change in environment changes our outlook. A few colorful paintings, throws, pillows, or curtains can make a delightful change in the mood of a room. Stick with light, bright, or pastel colors. Avoid dark, dull colors such as grey, brown, and black. At times these colors are the trend, yet their effect can pull your energy down. If you do use them, add white or ivory trims and light furniture and accessories.

Any color can be found in a wide variety of hues. For example, yellow can vary from a pale butter, summer lemon, banana mania, dandelion, sunglow, goldenrod, or gold. Add a little red or blue tint and it moves to an even wider palette.

Consider repainting walls with colorful, non-toxic paint. Even repainting a single wall can shift the mood of a room. Most paint departments provide color palette schemes to help select pleasing color combinations and accents. You can also create a color scheme by using colors found in one of your paintings, curtains, rugs, or pillows. Take a sample with you to help match colors.

Rearrange your furniture.

Rearranging your surroundings will stir up the energy in your home. Consider learning a few Feng Shui or Vaastu guidelines for ideas on new layouts.

Clear out stuff!

This practice ushers in a profound energy lift.

Clean out unwanted stuff to create space in your life. Space brings a higher vibration. Everything you own holds a vibration. Any item you aren't using, or that doesn't work right anymore, or that has an unpleasant connection with your past, needs to go! You'll be amazed at the renewed energy and clarity you experience when releasing these items from your environment! *(Details at end of book)*

Open blinds and curtains.

Maybe you want to hole up in your cave to lick your wounds, but isn't it better to heal them? Health and wellness require light. Even on cloudy days, the sun's rays penetrate through. Let it into your home. If you are concerned about privacy, hang white sheers which allow in the light while filtering what others can see from outside.

Air out your home.

At least once a week, bundle up and open the windows for 15-30 minutes to let fresh air flow through the house. Indoor air becomes polluted, depressing our mood and immune system.

Grow plants and herbs indoors, utilizing full spectrum bulbs or grow-lights.

You may become interested in a specific species of plant and enjoy learning about it. Some plants, such as African Violets, bloom and are pretty yet require attentive care.

If you don't have a green thumb, consider growing Golden Pothos vine. It is the easiest indoor plant to grow and it can be found in most floral sections of grocery or department stores. Pothos doesn't require as much light a many other houseplants. In fact, it does not like direct sun that is shining through a window. (But please don't place it in a windowless room and expect it to live!) It is usually grown in soil, but my mother grew many of her plants in water, and I do as well. Place cuttings in a vase of spring water (free of fluoride and chlorine). I add a few drops of liquid plant food to the water every few weeks. As your vine grows, you can arrange it in interesting ways, or cut it back, placing cuttings in water which will root quickly and expand your plant décor.

Flowers, flowers, flowers!

Place vases of flowers around your home. If finances

are an issue, many grocers and floral shops have discounted flowers that are several days old which still look beautiful. Thrift stores have a variety of interesting vases. Studies show that flowers boost your mood and reduce stress. And yes, flowers are for men, too!

Incense, Candles, and Essential Oil Diffusers

Environmental smells influence the subconscious, so treat your home to scents that are pleasing, mood-lifting, or comforting. Consider natural scents such as bergamot, citrus scents, clary sage, lavender, sandalwood, myrrh, frankincense, jasmine, and vanilla.

Purchase quality products. Incense sticks and cones that are made from pulverized resins and herbs provide the healing benefits you seek. Cheap incense which is made from pressed charcoal or sawdust dipped into perfume is less effective.

Use candles made from sustainable soy or other vegetable oils and infused with essential oils. Avoid paraffin candles scented with chemical perfumes which emit particulate matter. Go natural whenever possible. While the cost of natural products may be slightly more, they offer authentic healing benefits.

Salt Lamps.

Place these natural lamps in the main rooms you frequent – their negative ions are mood lifters. I can't speak highly enough about these beautiful lamps. They help remove toxins from the environment, offering a soft and cheerful light.

We moved into a new condominium, and I immediately became ill from toxic gasses releasing from the new paint, carpet, and cabinets. I was working long hours at the time and came home from work exhausted, only to be overwhelmed with toxins. I began to feel depressed and trapped. Every time I meditated, I asked for guidance on how to heal. A few weekends later, I attended a health fair. Walking down an aisle, I began to sense a warm, welcoming energy. I felt much lighter! Curious, I followed the sensation, and it led me to a booth that was set up with a row of salt lamps. I learned they were healing, purifying, and soothing. I immediately purchased three and set them up around the house. Within a few days, I began to feel better. Our house plants, which had been absorbing the toxins, also began to look healthier.

The effect of salt lamps is subtle, but benefits will accumulate over time.

Watch or listen to uplifting, motivating, and intellectually expanding media.

Movies, videos, podcasts, and documentaries offer fresh insights and inspiration.

Read uplifting and inspirational books.

Holding an uplifting book in hand is a comforting visceral experience. You can highlight areas of interest, make notes in the margin, and stick in copies of articles on similar subjects for future reference. Consider books on self-help or inspiring biographies of people who surmounted hardship.

Listen to upbeat, inspirational music.

Whistle! Drum on the countertop, tables, or washer. Sing! Don't worry about being on tune! Dance! Leap, twirl, reach, stomp, shimmy, liberate your soul through the magic of music! (*Also see "Music" chapter*)

Practice healing ceremonies.

There are a multitude of healing ceremonies you can conduct in your home. Smudging, bells, singing bowls, chanting, drumming, Vedic fire ceremony, pleasing scents, cleanliness, and organization, can all help create an environment supportive of self-awareness and self-assurance.

Agnihotra Healing Ceremony

Agnihotra, a profound Vedic fire ceremony, is performed at sunrise and sunset to create a home and neighborhood environment of peace, tranquility, and clarity.

Agnihotra is a simple process, yet a little more complex than many suggestions offered here. However, it has been scientifically proven to significantly decrease depression for the one who performs the ceremony as well as anyone within a two-mile radius. What could that mean to you?

(Agnihotra details at end of book)

12

Activities

If you do what you've always done,
you'll get what you've always got.
- Henry Ford

Choose one activity that is listed thus far and commit to its practice for 3 weeks.

Get out of your comfort zone.

Do something you've never done before. Climb out of your rut. Expand your experience. New experiences help break down old ways of thinking and introduce new possibilities.

Casey lost both his mother and his wife to cancer within a year. He felt lost and unsure of life. On a cloudy January Saturday, he was walking to buy cigarettes when he heard the melancholy music of a Spanish guitar and delighted laughter drifting out from a restaurant.

It was lunchtime, and he was hungry, but he'd never had Mexican food. He suddenly remembered that years ago he'd had a neighbor who played the

Spanish guitar, but he'd never heard anyone play one since. The smells and sounds drifting out of the restaurant were comforting. Remembering a conversation that I'd had with him about getting out of his comfort zone, he took a deep breath, opened the door, and walked in.

Seating himself at a booth, when the server asked for his order, he confessed, "I don't know anything about this kind of food."

Immediately, a couple in the next booth offered advice. The woman insisted, "Try the enchiladas and ask for mild sauce. But careful, you'll get addicted to them!" Her husband shook his head and said, "Naah, try a plate of sizzling fajitas!"

Laughing, Casey asked for descriptions of each, and conversation ensued. By the end of his meal (he ordered fajitas), they had invited him to a niece's birthday party that evening. He went and when the extended family learned of his recent tragedy, they welcomed him into their fold.

That's been seven years ago. Casey has since remarried, his new "family" attended his wedding, and they continue a close relationship.

Start new, creative projects.

Experiment with new hobbies, crafts, or sports.

Teach a free (or for donations) class on a hobby you enjoy.

Teaching others will connect you with like-minded

people and reinforce your self-confidence. And remember that you don't need to be an expert to teach. You only need to be eager to share and to know a little more than those who learn from you.

Cook or bake new recipes.

Try baking with one of the new flours such as spelt or einkorn. Choose a culture and experiment with their cuisine. Invite friends to join you.

Travel.

Go somewhere new. Get out of usual routine, even if it is only in another city or local area.

Eat out at new restaurants.

Try a new cuisine! Venture into another area of your town or community, or drive to another city.

Go to the library.

Today's libraries are totally different than a decade ago. You'll not only find books, but videos, CDs, podcasts, computers with free WIFI, 3D printers, genealogy records, seminars, and welcoming librarians who will answer any question. If all you do is sit at a table or in a comfy chair to read, you'll be out in the community and into the flow of energy that helps relieve a sense of isolation.

Intentionally help other people.

Get your mind off your own woes. Every day intentionally look for an opportunity to help someone, share information, or volunteer. Soup kitchens are wonderful place to help and recognize how fortunate you are. Gather warm socks, mufflers, food bars, other essentials for homeless people and distribute.

When you move out of your comfort zone to try something different, you never know what might be waiting. At the very least, you have stirred up possibilities.

13

Music

Music gives a soul to the universe,
wings to the mind, flight to the imagination,
and life to everything.
- Plato

Listen to music that either helps process depression or raises it to a higher vibration.

Science has shown that music creates vibrations that can either harmonize and raise your vibration, or create disharmony and energetic distress.

Sometimes, it does help to listen to music that "identifies" with your depression. As you feel it more deeply, it helps you access emotions so you can release them. But don't reside there. Process and then move on to music that lifts your spirits.

When processing through a traumatic time in my life, I constantly listened to sad music which spoke to what I was feeling. It helped me cry which released my angst. Once a crying session finished, I shifted to listening to positive, uplifting music with tones that nurtured and soothed. Over time, my despair lessened, to be replaced by hope. Following this flow, I slowly stopped listening to sad music which stirred up pain, instead continuing to focus on uplifting music. Eventually, along with other methods described in this book, my trauma dissolved into a sad memory that no longer influences my current life.

If you need energized, listen to motivating, inspiring music. For calm and reassurance, consider listening to music that is 432 Hz frequency. Because this is the frequency of nature, our body immediately relaxes.

Binaural beat therapy is also being researched for its healing benefits. Listened to on earphones, each ear hears a slightly different tone which the brain perceives as one. It is purported to help synchronize the right and left sides of the brain, offering healing and tranquility.

YouTube videos provide a wide variety of these types of music.

Chant or sing prayers and affirmations.

Prayers and chants in multiple traditions have demonstrated the ability to calm, energize, heal, transform, and shift brain patterns. Consistent repetition of high-vibration sounds elicits positive, empowering energetic influences. Onc such mantra is the Gayatri, which has been chanted for thousands of years. With repetition, its resonance nurtures the chanter's mind and body. *(Details at end of book)*

Join a community choir.

If you're not into big groups and weekly practices, get together with others to sing for fun. Gather friends to go out for a night of karaoke.

Join the local theater.

You can act, construct scenery, paint, do make-up, or help with wardrobe.

Learn to play a musical instrument.

Playing an instrument has been shown to reduce stress, increase patience, use almost every part of the brain, increase creativity, and strengthen confidence. Sharing music with friends enhances self-esteem and releases endorphins. Jam with other musicians or gather together your own band.

14

Self-Actualization and Spiritual

You yourself, as much as anybody in the entire universe, deserve your love and affection.
- Buddha

Any practice that honors yourself is a spiritual practice.

Any practice that honors someone else is a spiritual practice.

The human condition is not separate from the spiritual. A human being is spirit manifested into form, enlivened with purpose.

Every circumstance is an opportunity to transcend the human condition and apply spiritual principles.

The state of your consciousness in any circumstance determines your experience of it and how it is resolved.

Seek to live in the highest way you know.

Forgive yourself for mistakes. Learn from them (gain wisdom). Look for ways to apply your new wisdom.

Assist those around you to do the same.

Meditate or pray daily. Make a connection with something "greater" that reminds you of your wholeness.

Approach all circumstances with a neutral point of view. Hold no expectations or pre-conceived ideas. Observe with a calm mind that holds no opinions. Allow the situation to speak for itself and then make choices based on the best outcome for all involved.

Stay tuned in to "higher thinking" through a daily connection with inspirational videos, podcasts, articles, and books.

You are a soul, an immortal being of pure energy that is currently having a human experience. It's time to stop making choices as if you are "only a human". Be *you* at your highest and best.

Spiritualize your humanity.

Final Words

❖Act as if you are not depressed.

Make choices as if you are feeling good about yourself and life. *This is not being fake.* This is expressing the truth of your authentic self that is smothered beneath heavy layers of conditioned behaviors, old habits of thinking, and chronic hopelessness.

Who would you be if you were not depressed? How would you behave during any given day? What choices would you make? Would you get out more often? Smile more? Encourage other people? Take walks?

For which of the above solutions did you automatically say, "I wish I felt like it, but I just can't do that," because you are currently depressed? *Choose one and do it anyway.* How can acting that way be any worse than where you are now – stuck in depression?

❖Remember, act from what *works* instead of how you currently *feel*.

❖Constructive action creates more positive feedback.

❖Positive feedback releases serotonin.

❖Serotonin improves your mood and sense of self-worth.

❖Intentionally placing yourself into a constructive and positive cycle moves your energy and mind toward wholeness and self-fulfillment.

This is your life. Lead it!

15

Emotion Vibration Chart

*When one door of happiness closes, another opens;
but often we look so long at the closed door that we do
not see the one which has been opened for us.*
– Helen Keller

You are not your emotions. You are the one who experiences them.

Emotions are a precious and valuable feedback mechanism to help you navigate life. Observe them, learn from them, and then take charge.

Intentional Application Steps

1. Seek activities, books, articles, music, and videos to experience emotions in the upper five levels.

2. Avoid engaging in activities that increase or deepen emotions in the lower five levels.

The top five levels on the chart represent ascending levels of positivity, healing, and self-fulfillment.

The bottom five levels represent descending levels of negativity, dis-ease, and personal despair.

Emotional Vibration Chart

Appreciation, Blissful, Empowered, Freedom, Joy, Love, Passion

Compassion, Courage, Gratitude, Happiness, Spiritual Connection

Confident, Enthusiastic, Inspired, Open-Hearted, Responsible, Serene

At Ease, Eager, Empowered, Light-Hearted, Worthy

Acceptance, Contented, Encouraged, Faith, Hopeful, Optimistic, Positive

Boredom, Doubt, Disappointment, Insecurity, Lonely, Rejection

Blame, Frustration, Impatience, Irritation, Pessimism, Worry

Anger, Hatred, Fear, Judgement, Rage, Revenge

Abandoned, Anxiety, Guilt, Jealous, Sad, Shame, Unloved, Unworthy

Apathy, Depression, Disempowered, Despair, Grief, Hopeless, Powerless

16

Breath of Fire

*The most common way people give up their power
is by thinking they don't have any.*
– Alice Walker

Why not start your day by tapping into your personal power center?

Breath of Fire is known as *Agni Sara Pranayama* in Sanskrit and is taught in yoga traditions.

While this process initially sounds complicated, once you get the hang of it, it flows easily.

In the Ayurvedic tradition, breathing exercises are called *pranayama* (life-force control). Working with the breath, you can learn how to move life force through your body to create specific benefits. If you struggle with learning Fire Breath, contact a local yoga studio or search online for drawings, photos, or videos of the process.

Benefits

- Builds internal body heat
- Encourages free flow of *prana* (life-force)
- Builds energy
- Detoxifies mind and body
- Balances brain functions
- Enhances clarity of thought
- Increases feelings of presence, self-awareness, and confidence
- Oxygenates the blood
- Relieves tension
- Helps maintain body rhythms

Instructions

Place your feet hip-width apart.

Bend forward with back straight, arms straight, with hands placed on thighs for support.

Breathe in and out through the nose:

Inhale deeply, filling the abdomen – which will extend out as if a filled balloon. Then exhale completely (exhalation will be longer), exhaling out that final bit of breath until it's emptied completely.

Optional: Use "Ujjayi Breath" upon exhalation. Constrict the back of your throat so breath is "squeezed" through. Hint: hold your throat as if saying "huuuuh" with a closed mouth.

Holding your breath, drop your head (as if to look at stomach) and pull abdominal area ("stomach") in and up as far as you can (abdomen will be concave, as if a vacuum sucked it empty). Release the breath, allowing your abdomen to extend fully again.

Repeat 5X at a minimum. 1-2 sets of 5 repetitions are sufficient.

Do in the morning on an empty stomach.

If done first thing, it stokes your physical and mental fire.

Helpful Resource: BanyanBotanicals.com. Online searches offer additional resources.

17

Gayatri Mantra Chant

*Chanting is a way of getting in touch with yourself.
It's an opening of the heart and letting go of the mind
and thoughts. It deepens the channel of grace,
and it's a way of being present in the moment.*
- Krishna Das

Sound vibration influences the vibration of everything around it, including our body's energy field, along with our mental and emotional states of being. The vibration created by this specific chant brings upliftment, healing, and inspiration.

Gayatri Mantra (Sacred Song) is sung in Sanskrit. It brings Divine, cosmic, and illuminating light energy into the mind and heart.

> Om Bhur Bhuvah Swaha
>
> Tat Savitur Varenyam
>
> Bhargo Devasya Dhimahi,
>
> Dhiyo Yo Nah Prachodayat

Translation (non-literal)

"Throughout all realms of experience, the essential nature of illuminating existence is the Beloved Creator. May all beings perceive, through subtle and meditative intellect, the magnificent brilliance of enlightened awareness."

Sanskrit chants are always sung in Sanskrit because it contains the precise, desired vibrational frequency.

A Few Online Resources

You can listen to Gayatri, sing along as you learn the words, and/or sing it on your own as you go about your daily activities.

Gayatri Mantra – Divine Light Chant

by Ellie Hadsall: 3:11 minutes.
A simple acapella version for listening and practicing. Right click on the video picture's "setting" icon and set on "loop" for continuous listening.
https://**www.youtube.com**/watch?v=oP5DShW6kVA

Gayatri Mantra

by Deva Premal: 2 hours.
This is a sophisticated musical version. Very pleasing.
 https://**www.youtube.com**/watch?v=BSmToj9VZ4s

Gayatri Mantra

by Suresh Wadkar: 1:43 minutes.
Enlivening, calming, East Indian version.
https://**www.youtube.com**/watch?v=SarlTxrAbIY

The Gayatri Mantra

(108 Peaceful Chants – New). 44 minutes.
Uploaded by TheBless4Ever. A pleasing group chant.
Deep and resonant.
https://**www.youtube.com**/watch?v=P26ZvKY--KY

18

Self Massage

With every act of self-care your authentic self gets stronger, and the critical, fearful mind gets weaker. Every act of self-care is a powerful declaration: "I am on my side, I am on my side, each day I am more and more on my own side."
- Susan Weiss Berry

Healing Self Massage is known as *Abhyanga* in Sanskrit and practiced in the Ayurvedic natural healing system.

Regular, gentle oiling of your entire body is soothing and nurturing. Our skin is the largest organ, and nerve endings connect it with our muscles, bones, and internal organs.

It is recommended to massage at least once a week.

Items you need:

- Massage oil. Oil should be organic and unrefined when possible.

  Neutral oils that can be used by anyone are

organic sunflower, coconut, jojoba, sweet apricot kernel, and almond. If you have allergies, look up information on these oils before choosing which to use. Massage oils can be purchased at health food stores or online. Ayurveda recommends different types of massage oil for different body types.

Two resources for oils recommended for body types are www.Ayurveda.com and www.BanyanBotanicals.com

If desired, you can add a few drops of essential oil to your bottle of oil. In addition to the essential oils recommended for depression in Chapter 6, consider trying lavender, rose, sandalwood, or vetiver.

- 8-oz plastic squeeze bottle with pouring lid, or small oil cruet

- Container for holding hot water to warm the oil (a baby bottle warmer works great, too)

- Flat plate/container to set your oil bottle on (a large, inverted lid works well here)

- Large sheet of plastic (half of a cheap shower liner or curtain is perfect)

- Old large bath towel or old beach towel (often found at thrift stores)

- Old bath towel to wipe off oil

- Old bath towel to dry off after showering

- Pair of synthetic (washable) flip flops

- Shower cap or wrapping scarf to hold up hair

- Space heater (optional)

- Grease-cutting dish soap or cleanser

Instructions

Set up in a room that can be kept warm.

> A warm bathroom is convenient, but another room can be used if the bathroom needs to be open for others to use.

Pour half a cup of oil into plastic bottle. Warm by placing in hot water. Let it get warm, but never hot.

As oil warms, lay down your plastic sheet so the oil doesn't soak into the floor.

> Label the "top side" of the sheet with a marker so you don't lay the oily side onto the floor with future use.

Place your large bath or beach towel on the plastic sheet.

Place your flip flops and wiping towel next to the plastic sheet.

If your hair needs protection, cover it with a shower cap or wrap up in a scarf.

Turn on small room heater if you get chilled easily.

Pouring a small amount of oil in your palm at a time, begin to apply it to your body

Apply with firm, slow strokes.

On arms and legs, apply in long strokes from the hands/feet toward the center of the body.

On joints, apply with a circular motion.

On abdomen, apply in circular motion, moving upward on the right, across the top and downward on the left (following the motion of your intestines)

Apply oil to the body in the following order:

Seated or standing - apply to face, neck, shoulders, arms, torso front, and back.

Standing - apply to pelvic area and hips.

Seated - apply to each leg. Complete by oiling your feet, including soles and toes.

As you apply the oil, thank your body for all it does for you.

Once a week, oil your scalp.

Pour oil into your hands or small amounts directly onto the scalp. Massage the oil in gently.

You can oil your scalp daily if you prefer, but because it requires washing and re-doing hair, many people choose not to.

Place a small amount of oil onto your little finger and gently apply inside the ears and nose.

Sit for at least 10 minutes after completing your oil-down.

During this time, you may want to meditate or lay down for a light nap.

Avoid using electronics which only serve to attack your nervous system. This is the time to clear and calm your nerves so you can feel nurtured and peaceful.

Towel oil off with an old towel (store it so that it doesn't get oil on other things).

Wearing the flip flops, *carefully* walk to shower/tub.

Enter the shower/tub *carefully* so you don't slip – *oily feet easily slide on a slick or wet surface.*

Shower or bathe with a very mild soap. (I use moisturizing shampoo.)

Dry off with an old towel.

After several washings, when you can no longer get all the oil out of this towel, you can use it as your sitting towel.

To store, fold your plastic sheet over in half so the oily sides face each other.

You can just fold your seating towel over with the sheet. Store along with your wiping towel and flip flops for future use.

I highly recommend to keep a bottle of grease-cutting dish soap or cleanser handy.

Pour soap or cleanser down the tub or shower drain and flush with hot water after you finish so your drain doesn't clog from accumulated oil.

This sounds complicated in the beginning but once you set up your supplies and process, it becomes routine.

Just as in learning a new skill such as playing the piano, after several times of practice, self-massage becomes natural. It's worth it. You are worth it.

Helpful Resource: BanyanBotanicals.com. Online searches offer additional resources.

19

Candle Gazing

*All the darkness in the world
cannot extinguish the light of a single candle.*
– Francis of Assisi

Fire gazing has been used in many cultures. The Sanskrit word *Trataka* (to look upon or to gaze), originates from the Ayurvedic healing and lifestyle tradition.

Benefits

- The candle flame helps fulfill the eyes and pineal glands need for sunlight.
- Calms the mind and provides inner peace and silence.
- Brings greater clarity in mind and improves decision-making ability.
- Helps to overcome mental, behavioral, and emotional ailments.
- Provides stress relief and deep relaxation.
- Improves your concentration, intelligence, and memory.

- Serves as a meditation process or as preparation for meditation.
- Enhances self-esteem, self-confidence, patience, and willpower.
- Develops greater efficiency and productivity.
- Improves eyesight and vision.
- Deepens sleep and cures sleep related disorders such as headache, insomnia, nightmares, etc.

According to the Vedic text, *Gherand Samhita* (shloka 5.54), *Trataka* promotes clairvoyance and the perception of subtle manifestations.

Instructions

Light a candle and set it on a small, low table placed 3 to 4 feet in front of you.

Sit in a comfortable posture with the spine upright and the arms and shoulders relaxed.

Use any meditative posture which you can maintain *without any movement.*

Position the flame at the level of your eyes.

Face the candle directly without having to turn or strain your neck.

Arrange so the flame remains steady during the procedure.

Close windows, turn off fans, and close air conditioner or heater vents. Close the door if air flows in from other rooms.

Take a few deep breaths to relax.

Close the eyes and observe your breath for 5-6 breaths.

> The settled breath will steady your attention onto the candle.

Gaze at the flame.

> "Soften" your gaze to "observe" it, rather than intently staring at it.

> Look at any portion of the flame and avoid looking at the wick or candle or any portion other than the flame.

If distracted by outer events or thought, return your gaze to the flame.

Avoid moving body or head.

Avoid blinking as long as you can. At some point tears will begin to flow. When this occurs, close your eyes.

Try to hold the imprinted image of the flame in your mind and continue mentally gazing at it.

> Imagine it at the center of your forehead (between the brows – in front of the pineal gland)

If the image fades, open eyes and return gaze to the flame.

Repeat the process of observing until tears flow, closing eyes, and observing the after-image in area of pineal gland.

Repeat this cycle 2-3 times, or more as you prefer.

On completion of last cycle, open eyes and return attention to the room.

Sit quietly to re-orient yourself and then get up to proceed with the day.

Tips for Candle Gazing

Gazing is best practiced on an empty stomach during early-morning or late-evening immediately prior to bedtime. If you practice it during the daytime, make sure that the room is dark so that focusing on the flame is easier.

Try getting a decent sized flame by adjusting the size of the wick. It will help in achieving a better after-image of the flame and it will be easier to visualize it with improved concentration.

Do not strain your eyes while gazing on the flame. The eyes adjust naturally in due course of time, and it becomes easier to concentrate and gaze on the flame for longer periods of time.

20

Meditation on Breath

If you can breathe, you can meditate.
- Ellie

Meditation is a natural process that clears the mind of all mental fluctuations.

It is as natural as breathing, singing, dancing, praying, and visualizing.

It allows the mind to remain calm and open to insight and deepened understanding.

Meditation is the process of being mindful of your mental thoughts, releasing the constant mental and emotional chatter, and making space for peace, wisdom, and insight to arise.

The process itself is simple.

The challenge comes because as the mind quiets down, your current and dormant thoughts arise, seeking attention. This is to be expected. You will learn to handle these errant thoughts. They are not an interruption to your meditation; they are an integral part of it. With continued practice, they will begin to settle down.

Benefits

- Scientifically proven to bring benefits (you can find studies online.)
- Offers relaxation down to the cellular level
- Reduces stress and anxiety
- Creates even-mindedness in all circumstances
- Diffuses impatience and anger
- Increases self-assurance
- Minimizes dependence on outer events and people to bring self-fulfillment and joy
- Increases mental and emotional clarity
- Expands creativity
- Opens intuition
- Enhances positive outlook on life
- Diffuses and releases addictions
- Strengthens the immune system
- Promotes faster healing
- Establishes and maintains a clearer connection with the Source of life – whatever you perceive that to be.

Instructions

Find a quiet location. When possible, use the same location each time.

Your body and mind become conditioned to think "meditation!" when you sit in the same space.

Be Uninterrupted. Turn off phone, don't answer the

door, notify others to not interrupt you.

Get comfortable. Sit upright with a straight, but not stiff, spine; be alert but relaxed.

It's okay to lean back if it won't cause you to fall asleep. Accommodate your body. You can lay down if sitting isn't possible but adjust so you don't fall asleep.

Wear comfortable clothing. You may want a sweater or blanket, because your body temp may drop slightly.

I have a specific scarf I only use for meditation which I can wrap around my shoulders. I feel my body relax the moment I reach for it.

Close your eyes. You want to move your attention from outer life events to inner awareness.

Observe your breath. Simply observe your breath as it naturally moves in and out.

Allow it to flow naturally and just observe. It may be slow, rapid, irregular, smooth, shallow, deep ... anything is fine.

Breath flows as is necessary to support you. Breath knows what you need and adjusts accordingly. There is not a right or wrong way to breathe in this process – just allow it to "be" and observe it with your attention. If you find yourself holding breath, release it. If you "sigh" (breathing deeply and releasing), or yawn, simply observe.

The mind will wander, and thoughts will arise.

The moment you notice this, release the thought, and return attention to observing the breath. Your meditation will thus cycle back and forth.

Observe the Breath – Thought Arises –
Notice the Thought – Release the Thought –
Return to Observing the Breath.

At times you may follow a thought for a long time before remembering that you are meditating. This, too, is to be expected. When this happens simply follow the procedure by returning attention to the breath. Regardless of how mentally "busy" your meditation seems to be, your mind and body is benefitting.

Sit for 10-15 minutes a day.

If you struggle with 10 minutes in the beginning, practice for 5 minutes until that becomes easy and then lengthen your sittings in 5-minute increments. As you gain skill, sit for at least 20 minutes once or twice a day.

Move out of meditation slowly.

Your brain and body will have moved into a deeper state of consciousness. Your brain waves will have altered, and body processes slowed down. So, you need to adjust to outer surroundings slowly. If you come back quickly, it can cause headaches or jitteriness. If you are interrupted during meditation, handle the situation, and then move back into meditation so you can then move back out slowly.

No one session is transformational.
It is the accumulation of consistent daily practice
that creates the changes you seek.

There are many methods of meditation. Meditation on Breath is only one, but it is easily understood and practiced by millions across the globe.

My book "Meditation: A Journey to Self-Fulfillment" introduces and guides the reader through a multitude of meditation techniques from around the world, as well as helpful ways to prepare and center in for a more successful experience. Realistic solutions are offered for obstacles you may encounter.

Resource: Additional meditation information, podcasts, and a video demonstration by Ellie are available at www.EllieHadsall.com.

21

Agnihotra Vedic Fire Ceremony

…The yajnya confers fuller life and happiness. May this yajnya be performed everywhere. May the performer of the yajnya spread its knowledge. May the sacrificial fire keep us free from diseases…
- Yajur Veda: Chapter 1, Verse 22

Vedic Fire ceremony (*yajnya, havan,* or *homa)* is an ancient healing practice from the ancient Vedic tradition.

A small fire is burned in a small, inverted copper pyramid. Agnihotra is a specific simple fire ceremony for the purpose of removing harmful negative effects so that the natural harmony of the universe can express. It isn't just a gift to our planet; it is a multi-dimensional gift to the universe.

Fire is recognized as a major transforming agent in most cultures across our planet. The elements that are combined and burned may be changed by the fire into new chemical combinations.

Agni (fire) and *hotra* (fire pit or also one who

performs the ceremony of a fire) is one of the oldest of fire ceremonies. One of the fundamental healing fires, agnihotra's uniqueness is that it is practiced specifically at sunrise and sunset when a unique energy sweeps across the planet. As with all Vedic fire ceremonies, it has its own special features, purpose and results. Done with regularity, it creates an environment in which all living things receive healing, the atmosphere is purified, soil is re-enriched, and harmony reinstated.

Why do Agnihotra?

Have you ever desired to help heal the planet?

Have you wondered what you, as only one person, can do to make a difference?

Have you felt helpless as the environment appears to disintegrate around you, and wished you knew some positive action to take to help repair the damage done by humankind?

Agnihotra is a scientifically proven solution.

Anyone who wishes to heal themselves, others, animals, and plants, can do this fire ceremony. In doing so, one helps rebalance the planet's resources, removing toxins from the environment and replenishing the energy field of all manifested aspects, both animate and inanimate.

Anyone who has a sincere desire to live on this planet in a responsible manner can participate.

People from many cultures, countries, spiritual

traditions, and all ages are joining in this practice. Residents of Peru, Poland, the United States, Israel, Canada, Mexico, Hawaii, the Caribbean, Germany, Spain, West Indies, Australia, and South Africa are only a sample of those I personally know who are dedicated to this simple daily practice. Male or female, educated or uneducated, wealthy or poor, well respected or unknown to the eyes of the world, you can practice this.

Once you learn it and practice it with regularity you can begin to teach it to others. Its beauty is in its simplicity. You do the simple act and let the divine universe handle the results.

Benefits of Agnihotra

Agnihotra fire ceremony affects the planet through the effects of the fire itself, its smoke, and the resulting ash. Healing effects include but are not limited to:

People

Individuals who live in an area where regular Agnihotra fires are held experience the following: increased peace of mind, enhanced sense of well-being and calm, release of addictions, improved relationships, renewed vitality, faster healing of wounds, dissolution of toxins, and a reduction in frequency of illness and disease. Some scientific experiments indicate these reports are well founded.

Animals

Effects on animals parallels the effects of human

healing. Animals experience less disease, faster healing, calmer, more cooperative natures, and overall excellence of health. Disorders from years of neglect, herbicide and pesticide toxicity, antibiotics and other pharmaceuticals, and poor diet can all be reversed.

Plants

Plants grown in an Agnihotra environment grow exceptionally large and abundant fruit. Plants, and the resulting vegetables, fruit, nuts, or grains are healthy and more nutritious. Such plants do not need chemicals, artificial fertilizers, herbicides, or pesticides.

Soil that has been robbed of its vitality can be replenished with Agnihotra nutrients. Soil appears to retain moisture better and plants utilize moisture more efficiently. Science has demonstrated that Agnihotra causes a change in the cellular structure of the plant, creating a more efficient distribution of nutrients, including moisture.

We were excited to rent a newly remodeled house with a large backyard. Unfortunately, it was home to a diseased apple tree, dying apricot tree, and two-foot-high weeds. Having successfully grown organic gardens at former homes, we were determined to heal the trees and to create a serene space.

That spring, we set about digging a garden, only to discover that six to ten inches down into the soil, the entire yard was covered by a layer of old discarded roofing shingles. Our landlord promptly dug up the entire yard, removed the shingles and top dirt, and trucked in new, poor soil from an unknown source.

Knowing the healing properties of agnihotra, we set to work. Agnihotra ash was rubbed onto the tree trunks and larger lower branches. It was sprinkled around the base and watered in. We sprinkled agnihotra ash over the dirt as we worked in a minimal amount of cow manure and organic compost. My intent was to experiment with the agnihotra ash to investigate its potential. I set up a special area to perform agnihotra fires at as many sunrises and sunsets as I could work into my sixty-hour work week.

By the end of the summer our fruit trees were healed, and we were harvesting healthy organic produce. The following spring our apricot and apple trees were covered in blossoms and produced a plethora of fruit. We couldn't use it all, so invited friends to come over to pick the bounty. I planted rows of sunflowers that were supposed to grow four to five feet tall. By the end of the summer we had a sunflower forest branching up to fourteen feet high.

This is only one of many situations where agnihotra proved to be a powerful and nurturing support. My handbook, "Agnihotra-Havan on Earth", shares many fascinating stories of agnihotra's benefits.

Environment

Agnihotra purifies the atmosphere, soil, and water. It neutralizes radioactivity and toxins in the air. As it heals the plants and re-establishes balance in nature, the environment heals. The ash resulting from the fire, when added to water, has been shown to purify it of harmful effects. Toxic rivers where ash has been distributed have re-established a healthy eco system.

Healing Remedy

Agnihotra atmosphere and ash are mentioned in ancient Vedic texts as a means for prevention and cure of diseases. Agnihotra and other fire practices are included among other healing remedies as presented in Ayurveda (life-knowledge).

Thousands of people in different parts of the world report personal healings of a great variety of ailments by sitting in the smoke of the ceremony, some of which have been scientifically verified. The healing effects of Agnihotra are locked in the resulting purified ash which is then used as a natural healing remedy.

Psychotherapy

Agnihotra atmosphere removes stress and tension on the mind. It clears a space of the negative thought patterns that influence the mind. It allows one's innate intelligence to rise up into awareness. It opens the mind to creativity and possibilities. Agnihotra leads to greater clarity of thought, improves overall health, increases energy, and allows the mind to fill with love. This fire ceremony atmosphere promotes a deeper experience of meditation.

In addition to Agnihotra, there are other Vedic fire ceremonies.

A variety of fire ceremonies are offered for the purpose of clearing out an energy field, assisting in shifting into a new chosen reality, dissolving that which is no longer useful or wanted, creating, and manifesting the new into your life, releasing old attachments and relationships, joyful celebration, mental and emotional healing, assisting a group to experience compatible vibrations, and to re-awaken positive energetic force fields.

To Learn Agnihotra:

I have practiced and taught agnihotra for over 20 years. If you are interested in agnihotra as you read this, you might be receiving guidance to practice it. In addition to this specific ceremony practiced at sunrise and sunset, additional fire ceremonies can be practiced at any time of day. My 81-page handbook, *Agnihotra: Havan on Earth*: A simple and comprehensive guide to the practice of Agnihotra, a Vedic fire ceremony for personal and planetary healing, is available on Amazon.com. This is the first, and only, published handbook on the practice of this healing Vedic fire ceremony. Book includes photographs, personal stories of transformation, clear instructions, necessary resources, and over 60 FAQs! *Find more information, videos, and photos, at www.EllieHadsall.com*

22

Make Space for Joy

*The first step in crafting the life you want
is to get rid of everything you don't.*
- Joshua Becker

Depression is reinforced when your surroundings fail to lend support for your lifestyle.

As you look around your home and life, are there items that feel "heavy" to you? Maybe you feel uneasy each time you look at or handle them. Perhaps it's a gift someone gave you that you don't like, a couch you bought with your ex that you hang onto because you can't afford a new one, clothing that is still in good condition, but you never pull it out to wear anymore, or something that was perfect in the past but doesn't suit you in the present. Each "unwanted" item holds an energy cord that binds you. If your life is filled with enough of these cords, you are trapped, stuck, and feeling weighted down. It's time to cut through and toss off some of that weight. Free yourself up for more joy in life! Liberate yourself!

Instructions

1. Write down each item that you no longer want. Consider what causes pain or discomfort, or what is no longer useful to you. Don't forget to assess emotions or beliefs that no longer serve you.

2. For each item on your list, ask the following questions.

   - Do you need it?
   - Do you enjoy it?
   - Does it fit you?
   - Does it work right?
   - Does it fit your home?
   - Does it fit your budget?
   - Does it fit your ethics?
   - Does it fit your lifestyle?
   - Does it fit your personality?
   - Does it feel right?
   - Have you used it in the last six months?
   - Can you replace it if you need it in the future?
   - Does it help you feel more expansive?

3. If the answers are yes, keep it.

4. If any of the answers are "no", it's time to repair it or release it. You can give it away, donate it to a worthy organization, recycle it, sell it, or trade it.

5. If your issue is relationship oriented, it's time to act upon what you already suspect you need to do, take a relevant class, read self-help books, listen to informative podcasts, or seek counseling.

6. If the answers are mixed, or you are still unsure, pack it away somewhere for six months. If at the end of that time, you haven't dug it out again to use, release it.

Once you release only a few items, you'll notice how much lighter you feel!

The year following her divorce from an emotionally abusive husband, Melissa felt defeated. As my co-worker, we often discussed her situation over lunch. "I hate going home. Everything reminds me of my failed marriage."

I suggested she clear out items that held painful memories.

"That's my whole house!", she lamented, but the more she thought about it, the more she realized how much of their home had been his preferences and not hers. "I've always wanted a house that is light and cheerful!"

Melissa finally agreed to hold a yard sale. With the money earned from selling the couch, a dining set, queen bed, two chairs, and other unwanted household items, she could afford to look for what she wanted. In a few months she transformed her house from a dark, gloomy space into a light and airy home. Old drapes were replaced with gauzy curtains. A used, twin bedframe was painted white, and she covered her new bed with a multi-colored quilt her grandmother had made. Her old dresser got a fresh coat of white paint. A futon replaced the couch and served as a guest bed. With green plants, colorful pillows, and throws, her house was transformed from a gloomy, depressing hovel into a warm, inviting home. Refreshed by these changes, she went on to transform her wardrobe. The greatest benefit of all?

"As I sorted and tossed, I remembered the good times and the bad times," she said. "Cleaning out my house helped clean out my stuck emotions. I realized how I inwardly cringed each time I spotted something my ex had chosen. The first few days I cried constantly. But as I released things that held sad memories, I began to feel much lighter."

As we proceed through life, we accumulate stuff. My husband says, "We are born. We get stuff. We move stuff around. Then we die, leaving all that stuff behind."

Why waste time and energy with stuff that is no longer aligned with who you have become? As I help clients release stuff, they begin to relinquish old modes of thinking, self-judgment, and unworkability. Once liberated, you have fresh energy to create what you desire in the present.

***

In Summary...

You hold the key! You are the one and only person who can change your life.

If you picked up this book to read, you are either on

the cusp of desired change, or rapidly moving toward it.

Don't waste another precious day of your life being a victim, overwhelmed, trapped, helpless, insignificant, fearful, unloved, defenseless, or powerless.

You were born and are living for a reason. What you have to offer is needed by others.

Humanity kindly requests your full participation.

Blast through the morass of Winter Blues and raise yourself to a new level of beingness.

> *"I have always believed, and I still believe,*
> *that whatever good or bad fortune may come our way*
> *we can always give it meaning and transform it*
> *into something of value."*
> - Hermann Hesse

23

Author

Ellie Hadsall is an author, intuitive, minister, meditation leader, personal and spiritual mentor. During her career, she has served as an inspirational speaker and professional trainer in human relations, communication, and self-development. A daily meditator and leader of meditations for over 35 years, she is ordained in the Kriya tradition, with a focus on practical application of spiritual practices into daily life.

Ellie experienced a deep, lingering postpartum depression after the birth of her first child.

I was excited to welcome our firstborn into this world. My months of pregnancy were easy. I was healthy, active, and eager to learn mothering. I read every book I could find on childbirth and parenting and took classes with the La Leche League to learn how to breast feed.

Natural childbirth was not available in those years. My husband was a military officer, and I was cared for by military doctors who were his superiors. The night our daughter was born, the obstetrician delivered seven babies. Protocols were rigid and demanding. My water broke and was followed by eleven hours of dry labor. My husband was not allowed in my room during labor or in the delivery room. Breastfeeding was not supported. I struggled to maintain a positive outlook and barely managed to do so until a few weeks later when postpartum depression set in.

I switched from being an outgoing, enthusiastic, positive woman into a person I barely recognized. I felt ugly, unwanted, and insufficient. My former life had been filled with eagerness, goals, rich relationships, and joy.

Now, I faced each moment with a dread that I didn't recognize. My husband's loving reassurance rang empty because I didn't believe he saw the deep truth - that I was no longer the same person.

Having nowhere to turn for help, and determined that my child would have a happy, inspiring, productive mother, I acted from my former self, hiding my self-doubt from family and friends.

In time, my hormones adjusted, and my former self returned. Three years later we moved from Kansas to northern Indiana, where the Great Lakes form unique winter weather patterns. Winter days were shorter and winter skies were often grey. Snowfall was beautiful in those years, but soon the streets were lined with mountains of grey, dirty snow. I became desperate for sunshine. I remember one day driving down the street filled with panic. I felt as if I had to leave and drive southward to confirm to myself that somewhere the sun still existed. In that moment, I realized I had to find a way to change my perception of winter. Somehow, I needed to take charge of my life and conquer the winter blues. This began my diligent search for solutions.

I have suffered the deep emptiness and hopelessness of depression. This booklet includes many of the methods I used to survive and flourish until I healed. As time has passed, many have become integrated into my daily lifestyle. These practices have led me into a more advanced and self-confident expression of my Self.

If only a few suggestions help someone, then I have been successful in helping others find hope and peace.

Ellie's Books

Available on Amazon and other online bookstores.

ଚ **Pathwalker** ଓ

A Soul's Journey Through Parallel Lives
Cave Time Chronicles, Bk 1

Eleni is in her groove with an amazing relationship and fulfilling life until she is suddenly transported into an unknown existence. Struggling to survive, she can only depend upon two things: a fading memory of who she used to be, and an intangible presence she has always called "Source".

From a Reader: *This is the BEST...fiction book I have read in years. I could not put it down! The story is super engaging.*

❧ **Spiritdancer** ☙
A Soul's Journey Through Parallel Lives
Cave Time Chronicles, Bk 2

Quantum travel, wisdom trees, a fleeing gypsy caravan, cataclysmic war, a serene country refuge, healing herbs, life-threatening global disintegration, and a loyal wolf bring a new level of intensity as Eleni comes to terms with her dance through yet another parallel lifetime.

❧ **Meditation** ☙
A Journey to Self-Fulfillment
An Exploration of Meditation Techniques from Multiple Traditions, and Practical Steps to Apply Them Successfully in Your Life.

This handbook introduces techniques from multiple traditions and offers realistic and practical solutions to the challenges of mastering meditation.

❧ **Agnihotra: Havan on Earth** ☙
A simple and comprehensive guide to the practice of Agnihotra, a Vedic fire ceremony for personal and planetary healing.

This is the first, and only, published handbook on the practice of this healing Vedic fire ceremony. Book includes photographs, fascinating personal stories of transformation, clear instructions, resources, and over 60 FAQs.

Additional agnihotra information, videos, downloads, and photos at *EllieHadsall.com*

❧ **Conquering the Winter Blues** ☙

Over 60 Steps to Tackle Seasonal Affective Disorder and Depression. Encouraging and inspiring.

❧ **Foraging in a City Yard** ☙

Ellie grew up eating weeds and now shares their delicious benefits with family and community. This colorful book on backyard foraging includes photos, identification, nutritional benefits, and recipes of 26 common weeds found in cities across the globe.

Future Books

❧ **Snowtracker** ☙

A Soul's Journey Through Parallel Lives
Cave Time Chronicles, Bk 3
Look forward to our heroine's emergence into a strange, frozen world of swirling snow, unexpected companions, new insights, and life-threatening adventure.

More book information at *www.EllieHadsall.com*

www.ingramcontent.com/pod-product-compliance
Lightning Source LLC
Chambersburg PA
CBHW070719250726
48662CB00001B/486